Essential Oils
30 Essential Oil Shower Bombs

Table of content

Introduction

It was a long day at the office, or at the gym, or anywhere for that matter. You are hot, tired, and sore, just wanting to slip into something comfy and let the day wash off. If only there was a way to get you own personal spa treatment right there at home.

You spent hours poring over that idea for work. You put your heart and soul into it, and now you just want to relax and let it all melt away while you forget about the worries of the day in a nice, hot bath.

But bath bombs scare you. You have read the ingredient list, and you see they are full of chemicals and other things you can't even pronounce, which makes you nervous about using them. You spend so much time taking care of your health, you can't afford to dump it all down the drain in order to relax.

You just think if only you could make your own, everything would be better. You could pick and choose what you put into it, the scent you want it to be, and exactly what you hope to accomplish. Think of it as your own personal spa experience, and you get exactly what you want, when you want it.

This is the perfect idea for anyone that likes to be in control of their health, enjoy a nice relaxing bath after work, and gain all of the aromatherapy benefits of essential oils. This truly is the perfect situation for you to indulge in when you get home from a long day at work.

So what are you waiting for? You know you would love to indulge in the spa experience every day you could, and now, you can. You can have it all whenever you want, however you want. Think of it as your own little pampering for all that you do, better than the spa because it is personal and incredibly less expensive.

This is an all-around win for anyone that likes to be pampered and save money, as well as reap the incredible benefits for their health. You can have it all and then some, which is exactly what you are going to get with any one of these bath bombs.

Go ahead, indulge a little.

Chapter 1 – Getting Started: How to Make Your Bath Bomb

If you have ever used a bath bomb, you know they are a lot of fun to toss into the tub and watch fizz away into nothing. At the same time, the scent they release into the air is perfect for melting away any worries or any stress that day brought in.

In addition to that, you will see that your headaches, body aches, or any other pains that you may have will also melt away as your bomb fizzes its way into the tub.

With that in mind, however, if you have never made a bath bomb, you may wonder how you are able to get them into that hard ball that then fizzes its way into bathtub bliss for your enjoyment. Let me assure you, the answer is simple. A bath bomb is nothing more than a few ingredients that are combined in the right ratio to make the perfect bath buddy.

In the chapters to come, I am going to show you how to make your own bath bombs using the essential oils that you choose for the recipe, but you are going to use this same basic recipe to form each of the bombs. There is enough here to make several small bath bombs per batch, but if you want more, simply double the recipe.

Here are the basic ingredients you are going to need for your bath bombs

- 8 ounces baking soda

- 4 ounces corn starch

- 2 ounces Epsom salt (only the finest grained variety)

- Fine grained Himalayan sea salt

- 4 ounces citric acid

- Powdered sugar

- 1 ½ teaspoons carrier oil of your choice (I prefer to use coconut)

And, of course, the essential oils, but we are going to add those in later on. For each of the recipes, when you see the ingredient "bomb mix" this is what I am referring to. No matter what the recipe is, you are going to use this basic mix for the shaping and body of the bomb.

In addition to the ingredients you will need for the bombs, you are also going to need a few supplies

- **Wire whisk or wooden spoon (I prefer the whisk)**

- **Large bowl**

- **Baking sheet (or molds, if you prefer uniform size and shape)**

- **Towels (paper or otherwise, it's up to you)**

That's really all you need to make your bombs. The method is going to be the same for all of them, but we will get into that later on.

Remember to use carrier oil, not matter what kind it is

A lot of people like to use water in their bath bombs, but trust me, a carrier oil is your best friend. Some oils are harsh to come into contact with on your skin, and while you are using a light amount in your bath bombs, you never know what your own personal sensitivity is going to be like.

With that in mind, you need to use a carrier oil of some kind. It doesn't really matter what kind of carrier oil you use, although I would recommend coconut oil. Coconut oil is excellent for your skin, it's virtually unscented so you don't have to worry about it clashing with your essential oils, and it is inexpensive, so you don't have to worry about breaking the bank to get it.

Once you have all of your ingredients on hand, you are ready to begin, so let's get into it.

Chapter 2 – Weekend Bombs

Friday Night Bath Bombs

What you will need:

10 drops chamomile

10 drops rose

10 drops peppermint

Bomb mix

Directions:

Start by combining the dry ingredients in a bowl, then combine all of the wet ingredients in another bowl. I find that it is best to use the whisk for this part, though you may need to use the wooden spoon next.

Pour the wet ingredients into the dry ingredients and mix well. The ingredients are going to form a dough, so keep mixing. If it's too dry add in a bit of water, but be very careful not to add too much and ruin the bombs.

Use your hands dusted with powder sugar to form balls about the same size. You may make these as large or as small as you would like.

Let the bombs set on a baking sheet that has been lined with a towel. It is going to take roughly 24 hours for them to dry completely.

Wrap in tissue paper to store until use.

Pamper Yourself Bomb

What you will need:

10 drops rosemary

10 drops lemongrass

10 drops lavender

Bomb mix

Directions:

Start by combining the dry ingredients in a bowl, then combine all of the wet ingredients in another bowl. I find that it is best to use the whisk for this part, though you may need to use the wooden spoon next.

Pour the wet ingredients into the dry ingredients and mix well. The ingredients are going to form a dough, so keep mixing. If it's too dry add in a bit of water, but be very careful not to add too much and ruin the bombs.

Use your hands dusted with powder sugar to form balls about the same size. You may make these as large or as small as you would like.

Let the bombs set on a baking sheet that has been lined with a towel. It is going to take roughly 24 hours for them to dry completely.

Wrap in tissue paper to store until use.

Glory Goddess

What you will need:

10 drops goldenseal

10 drops patchouli

10 drops lavender

Bomb mix

Directions:

Start by combining the dry ingredients in a bowl, then combine all of the wet ingredients in another bowl. I find that it is best to use the whisk for this part, though you may need to use the wooden spoon next.

Pour the wet ingredients into the dry ingredients and mix well. The ingredients are going to form a dough, so keep mixing. If it's too dry add in a bit of water, but be very careful not to add too much and ruin the bombs.

Use your hands dusted with powder sugar to form balls about the same size. You may make these as large or as small as you would like.

Let the bombs set on a baking sheet that has been lined with a towel. It is going to take roughly 24 hours for them to dry completely.

Wrap in tissue paper to store until use.

Candlelight Sonata

What you will need:

10 drops tea tree

5 drops rose

5 drops cardamom

10 drops vetiver

Bomb mix

Directions:

Start by combining the dry ingredients in a bowl, then combine all of the wet ingredients in another bowl. I find that it is best to use the whisk for this part, though you may need to use the wooden spoon next.

Pour the wet ingredients into the dry ingredients and mix well. The ingredients are going to form a dough, so keep mixing. If it's too dry add in a bit of water, but be very careful not to add too much and ruin the bombs.

Use your hands dusted with powder sugar to form balls about the same size. You may make these as large or as small as you would like.

Let the bombs set on a baking sheet that has been lined with a towel. It is going to take roughly 24 hours for them to dry completely.

Wrap in tissue paper to store until use.

Wings of Xerxes

What you will need:

5 drops sandalwood

5 drops lemon

10 drops ravintsara

10 drops myrrh

Bomb mix

Directions:

Start by combining the dry ingredients in a bowl, then combine all of the wet ingredients in another bowl. I find that it is best to use the whisk for this part, though you may need to use the wooden spoon next.

Pour the wet ingredients into the dry ingredients and mix well. The ingredients are going to form a dough, so keep mixing. If it's too dry add in a bit of water, but be very careful not to add too much and ruin the bombs.

Use your hands dusted with powder sugar to form balls about the same size. You may make these as large or as small as you would like.

Let the bombs set on a baking sheet that has been lined with a towel. It is going to take roughly 24 hours for them to dry completely.

Wrap in tissue paper to store until use.

Chapter 3 – Aches and Pains Bath Bombs

The Winter Rose

What you will need:

10 drops wintergreen

10 drops peppermint

10 drops rose

Bomb mix

Directions:

Start by combining the dry ingredients in a bowl, then combine all of the wet ingredients in another bowl. I find that it is best to use the whisk for this part, though you may need to use the wooden spoon next.

Pour the wet ingredients into the dry ingredients and mix well. The ingredients are going to form a dough, so keep mixing. If it's too dry add in a bit of water, but be very careful not to add too much and ruin the bombs.

Use your hands dusted with powder sugar to form balls about the same size. You may make these as large or as small as you would like.

Let the bombs set on a baking sheet that has been lined with a towel. It is going to take roughly 24 hours for them to dry completely.

Wrap in tissue paper to store until use.

The Magic Mix

What you will need:

10 drops frankincense

10 drops bergamot

10 drops cedarwood

Bomb mix

Directions:

Start by combining the dry ingredients in a bowl, then combine all of the wet ingredients in another bowl. I find that it is best to use the whisk for this part, though you may need to use the wooden spoon next.

Pour the wet ingredients into the dry ingredients and mix well. The ingredients are going to form a dough, so keep mixing. If it's too dry add in a bit of water, but be very careful not to add too much and ruin the bombs.

Use your hands dusted with powder sugar to form balls about the same size. You may make these as large or as small as you would like.

Let the bombs set on a baking sheet that has been lined with a towel. It is going to take roughly 24 hours for them to dry completely.

1

Wrap in tissue paper to store until use.

Fizz Your Cares Away

What you will need:

10 drops grapefruit

10 drops lemon

5 drops lemongrass

5 drops orange

Directions:

Start by combining the dry ingredients in a bowl, then combine all of the wet ingredients in another bowl. I find that it is best to use the whisk for this part, though you may need to use the wooden spoon next.

Pour the wet ingredients into the dry ingredients and mix well. The ingredients are going to form a dough, so keep mixing. If it's too dry add in a bit of water, but be very careful not to add too much and ruin the bombs.

Use your hands dusted with powder sugar to form balls about the same size. You may make these as large or as small as you would like.

Let the bombs set on a baking sheet that has been lined with a towel. It is going to take roughly 24 hours for them to dry completely.

Wrap in tissue paper to store until use.

The Dancing Man

What you will need:

10 drops ylang ylang

10 drops patchouli

10 drops petitgrain

Bomb mix

Directions:

Start by combining the dry ingredients in a bowl, then combine all of the wet ingredients in another bowl. I find that it is best to use the whisk for this part, though you may need to use the wooden spoon next.

Pour the wet ingredients into the dry ingredients and mix well. The ingredients are going to form a dough, so keep mixing. If it's too dry add in a bit of water, but be very careful not to add too much and ruin the bombs.

Use your hands dusted with powder sugar to form balls about the same size. You may make these as large or as small as you would like.

Let the bombs set on a baking sheet that has been lined with a towel. It is going to take roughly 24 hours for them to dry completely.

Wrap in tissue paper to store until use.

Kisses and Cashmere

What you will need:

10 drops vanilla

10 drops sandalwood

10 drops rose

Bomb mix

Directions:

Start by combining the dry ingredients in a bowl, then combine all of the wet ingredients in another bowl. I find that it is best to use the whisk for this part, though you may need to use the wooden spoon next.

Pour the wet ingredients into the dry ingredients and mix well. The ingredients are going to form a dough, so keep mixing. If it's too dry add in a bit of water, but be very careful not to add too much and ruin the bombs.

Use your hands dusted with powder sugar to form balls about the same size. You may make these as large or as small as you would like.

Let the bombs set on a baking sheet that has been lined with a towel. It is going to take roughly 24 hours for them to dry completely.

Wrap in tissue paper to store until use.

Chapter 4 – Stress Melting Bath Bombs

Happy Days

What you will need:

10 drops ylang ylang

10 drops vanilla

10 drops lavender

Bomb mix

Directions:

Start by combining the dry ingredients in a bowl, then combine all of the wet ingredients in another bowl. I find that it is best to use the whisk for this part, though you may need to use the wooden spoon next.

Pour the wet ingredients into the dry ingredients and mix well. The ingredients are going to form a dough, so keep mixing. If it's too dry add in a bit of water, but be very careful not to add too much and ruin the bombs.

Use your hands dusted with powder sugar to form balls about the same size. You may make these as large or as small as you would like.

Let the bombs set on a baking sheet that has been lined with a towel. It is going to take roughly 24 hours for them to dry completely.

Wrap in tissue paper to store until use.

A Summer Picnic

What you will need:

10 drops wild orange

10 drops wheatgrass

5 drops lemongrass

5 drops orange

Bomb mix

Directions:

Start by combining the dry ingredients in a bowl, then combine all of the wet ingredients in another bowl. I find that it is best to use the whisk for this part, though you may need to use the wooden spoon next.

Pour the wet ingredients into the dry ingredients and mix well. The ingredients are going to form a dough, so keep mixing. If it's too dry add in a bit of water, but be very careful not to add too much and ruin the bombs.

Use your hands dusted with powder sugar to form balls about the same size. You may make these as large or as small as you would like.

Let the bombs set on a baking sheet that has been lined with a towel. It is going to take roughly 24 hours for them to dry completely.

Wrap in tissue paper to store until use.

Fairly Fairies

What you will need:

5 drops sunflower

10 drops rose

5 drops lilac

5 drops lemongrass

5 drops vanilla

Bomb mix

Directions:

Start by combining the dry ingredients in a bowl, then combine all of the wet ingredients in another bowl. I find that it is best to use the whisk for this part, though you may need to use the wooden spoon next.

Pour the wet ingredients into the dry ingredients and mix well. The ingredients are going to form a dough, so keep mixing. If it's too dry add in a bit of water, but be very careful not to add too much and ruin the bombs.

Use your hands dusted with powder sugar to form balls about the same size. You may make these as large or as small as you would like.

Let the bombs set on a baking sheet that has been lined with a towel. It is going to take roughly 24 hours for them to dry completely.

Wrap in tissue paper to store until use.

Cricket's Song

What you will need:

10 drops myrrh

10 drops goldenseal

5 drops lemon

5 drops peppermint

Bomb mix

Directions:

Start by combining the dry ingredients in a bowl, then combine all of the wet ingredients in another bowl. I find that it is best to use the whisk for this part, though you may need to use the wooden spoon next.

Pour the wet ingredients into the dry ingredients and mix well. The ingredients are going to form a dough, so keep mixing. If it's too dry add in a bit of water, but be very careful not to add too much and ruin the bombs.

Use your hands dusted with powder sugar to form balls about the same size. You may make these as large or as small as you would like.

Let the bombs set on a baking sheet that has been lined with a towel. It is going to take roughly 24 hours for them to dry completely.

Wrap in tissue paper to store until use.

Whimsical Wishes

What you will need:

10 drops neroli

10 drops bergamot

5 drops pine

5 drops cedarwood

Directions:

Start by combining the dry ingredients in a bowl, then combine all of the wet ingredients in another bowl. I find that it is best to use the whisk for this part, though you may need to use the wooden spoon next.

Pour the wet ingredients into the dry ingredients and mix well. The ingredients are going to form a dough, so keep mixing. If it's too dry add in a bit of water, but be very careful not to add too much and ruin the bombs.

Use your hands dusted with powder sugar to form balls about the same size. You may make these as large or as small as you would like.

Let the bombs set on a baking sheet that has been lined with a towel. It is going to take roughly 24 hours for them to dry completely.

Wrap in tissue paper to store until use.

Chapter 5 – A Drop of the Joy Bomb Bath Bombs

The Stars and Stripes

What you will need:

10 drops agar

10 drops camphor

5 drops rose

5 drops cardamom

Bomb mix

Directions:

Start by combining the dry ingredients in a bowl, then combine all of the wet ingredients in another bowl. I find that it is best to use the whisk for this part, though you may need to use the wooden spoon next.

Pour the wet ingredients into the dry ingredients and mix well. The ingredients are going to form a dough, so keep mixing. If it's too dry add in a bit of water, but be very careful not to add too much and ruin the bombs.

Use your hands dusted with powder sugar to form balls about the same size. You may make these as large or as small as you would like.

Let the bombs set on a baking sheet that has been lined with a towel. It is going to take roughly 24 hours for them to dry completely.

Wrap in tissue paper to store until use.

Sun, Moon, and Shine

What you will need:

10 drops carrot seed

5 drops orange

5 drops chamomile

10 drops vanilla

Bomb mix

Directions:

Start by combining the dry ingredients in a bowl, then combine all of the wet ingredients in another bowl. I find that it is best to use the whisk for this part, though you may need to use the wooden spoon next.

Pour the wet ingredients into the dry ingredients and mix well. The ingredients are going to form a dough, so keep mixing. If it's too dry add in a bit of water, but be very careful not to add too much and ruin the bombs.

Use your hands dusted with powder sugar to form balls about the same size. You may make these as large or as small as you would like.

Let the bombs set on a baking sheet that has been lined with a towel. It is going to take roughly 24 hours for them to dry completely.

Wrap in tissue paper to store until use.

It's a Holiday

What you will need:

10 drops ginger

10 drops cinnamon bark

10 drops peppermint

Bomb mix

Directions:

Start by combining the dry ingredients in a bowl, then combine all of the wet ingredients in another bowl. I find that it is best to use the whisk for this part, though you may need to use the wooden spoon next.

Pour the wet ingredients into the dry ingredients and mix well. The ingredients are going to form a dough, so keep mixing. If it's too dry add in a bit of water, but be very careful not to add too much and ruin the bombs.

Use your hands dusted with powder sugar to form balls ab

out the same size. You may make these as large or as small as you would like.

Let the bombs set on a baking sheet that has been lined with a towel. It is going to take roughly 24 hours for them to dry completely.

Wrap in tissue paper to store until use.

Splashes and Sashes

What you will need:

10 drops clary sage

5 drops rosewood

5 drops cedarwood

10 drops tea tree

Bomb mix

Directions:

Start by combining the dry ingredients in a bowl, then combine all of the wet ingredients in another bowl. I find that it is best to use the whisk for this part, though you may need to use the wooden spoon next.

Pour the wet ingredients into the dry ingredients and mix well. The ingredients are going to form a dough, so keep mixing. If it's too dry add in a bit of water, but be very careful not to add too much and ruin the bombs.

Use your hands dusted with powder sugar to form balls about the same size. You may make these as large or as small as you would like.

Let the bombs set on a baking sheet that has been lined with a towel. It is going to take roughly 24 hours for them to dry completely.

Wrap in tissue paper to store until use.

Spring Fever

What you will need:

10 drops lilac

10 drops davana

10 drops eucalyptus

Bomb mix

Directions:

Start by combining the dry ingredients in a bowl, then combine all of the wet ingredients in another bowl. I find that it is best to use the whisk for this part, though you may need to use the wooden spoon next.

Pour the wet ingredients into the dry ingredients and mix well. The ingredients are going to form a dough, so keep mixing. If it's too dry add in a bit of water, but be very careful not to add too much and ruin the bombs.

Use your hands dusted with powder sugar to form balls about the same size. You may make these as large or as small as you would like.

Let the bombs set on a baking sheet that has been lined with a towel. It is going to take roughly 24 hours for them to dry completely.

Wrap in tissue paper to store until use.

Chapter 6 – Because You Need Pampered Bath Bombs

A Day at the Beach

What you will need:

10 drops eucalyptus

10 drops fir

5 drops orange

5 drops lemon

Bomb mix

Directions:

Start by combining the dry ingredients in a bowl, then combine all of the wet ingredients in another bowl. I find that it is best to use the whisk for this part, though you may need to use the wooden spoon next.

Pour the wet ingredients into the dry ingredients and mix well. The ingredients are going to form a dough, so keep mixing. If it's too dry add in a bit of water, but be very careful not to add too much and ruin the bombs.

Use your hands dusted with powder sugar to form balls about the same size. You may make these as large or as small as you would like.

Let the bombs set on a baking sheet that has been lined with a towel. It is going to take roughly 24 hours for them to dry completely.

Wrap in tissue paper to store until use.

Suntan Lotion and Bikinis

What you will need:

10 drops grapefruit

10 drops jasmine

5 drops vanilla

5 drops juniper

Bomb mix

Directions:

Start by combining the dry ingredients in a bowl, then combine all of the wet ingredients in another bowl. I find that it is best to use the whisk for this part, though you may need to use the wooden spoon next.

Pour the wet ingredients into the dry ingredients and mix well. The ingredients are going to form a dough, so keep mixing. If it's too dry add in a bit of water, but be very careful not to add too much and ruin the bombs.

Use your hands dusted with powder sugar to form balls about the same size. You may make these as large or as small as you would like.

Let the bombs set on a baking sheet that has been lined with a towel. It is going to take roughly 24 hours for them to dry completely.

Wrap in tissue paper to store until use.

Beach Towels

What you will need:

10 drops parsley

10 drops patchouli

5 drops lavender

5 drops bergamot

Bomb mix

Directions:

Start by combining the dry ingredients in a bowl, then combine all of the wet ingredients in another bowl. I find that it is best to use the whisk for this part, though you may need to use the wooden spoon next.

Pour the wet ingredients into the dry ingredients and mix well. The ingredients are going to form a dough, so keep mixing. If it's too dry add in a bit of water, but be very careful not to add too much and ruin the bombs.

Use your hands dusted with powder sugar to form balls about the same size. You may make these as large or as small as you would like.

Let the bombs set on a baking sheet that has been lined with a towel. It is going to take roughly 24 hours for them to dry completely.

Wrap in tissue paper to store until use.

Elegance Divine

What you will need:

5 drops marjoram

5 drops Melissa

10 drops vanilla

10 drops myrrh

Bomb mix

Directions:

Start by combining the dry ingredients in a bowl, then combine all of the wet ingredients in another bowl. I find that it is best to use the whisk for this part, though you may need to use the wooden spoon next.

Pour the wet ingredients into the dry ingredients and mix well. The ingredients are going to form a dough, so keep mixing. If it's too dry add in a bit of water, but be very careful not to add too much and ruin the bombs.

Use your hands dusted with powder sugar to form balls about the same size. You may make these as large or as small as you would like.

Let the bombs set on a baking sheet that has been lined with a towel. It is going to take roughly 24 hours for them to dry completely.

Wrap in tissue paper to store until use.

Shine and Dine

What you will need:

10 drops star anise

5 drops tangerine

5 drops parsley

5 drops rose

5 drops myrrh

Bomb mix

Directions:

Start by combining the dry ingredients in a bowl, then combine all of the wet ingredients in another bowl. I find that it is best to use the whisk for this part, though you may need to use the wooden spoon next.

Pour the wet ingredients into the dry ingredients and mix well. The ingredients are going to form a dough, so keep mixing. If it's too dry add in a bit of water, but be very careful not to add too much and ruin the bombs.

Use your hands dusted with powder sugar to form balls about the same size. You may make these as large or as small as you would like.

Let the bombs set on a baking sheet that has been lined with a towel. It is going to take roughly 24 hours for them to dry completely.

Wrap in tissue paper to store until use.

Conclusion

There you have it, everything you need to know to make your own bath bombs, and how you can use them to make your day more relaxing and a lot less hectic. Imagine what kind of a day you would have if you knew you were going to come home to a nice hot bath as soon as you got back.

All of the stress that you feel pent up inside you would melt away, and you would be able to indulge in a richness that is fit for a king. Think of the healthy benefits you are going to gain when you skip out on those chemicals that like to creep into the everyday things that you enjoy, and think of the mental benefits you are going to gain from relaxing in a hot bath at the end of a long day.

It doesn't seem to matter what kind of job you have, how old you are, or how many hours you worked that day. Just knowing you are going to come home to a nice hot bath is enough to make your day go by quickly, and make it seem a lot better as it does. Feeling tight and cramped at the end of the day? You have a bomb for that.

Feeling as stressed and like you can't do anymore of this? You have a bomb for that. Just craving a nice, fresh smell as you relax in your bath and melt all of your worries away? You have a bomb for that, too. When you stop to think about it you have a bomb for anything you want, and anything that happens to you in your day is completely manageable because of that fact.

No more anxiety, no more muscle tension, no more stress that just hangs onto your life well into the night. With your selection of bath bombs, you have what you need to get through any day, and put any problem to rest as soon as it pops up.

This book is going to be your guide to a less stress, no mess life. Let go of the little things that like to creep into your day, and you will feel so much better as you head to bed. This is why you can wake up feeling rested and ready to start the next day as it comes.

And the secret is simple, just relax in your bath with a personalized bomb. Your own little spa getaway, right in the middle of your home.

www.ingramcontent.com/pod-product-compliance
Lightning Source LLC
Chambersburg PA
CBHW071125280526
45787CB00003B/1166